Gluten Free Diet for Beginners

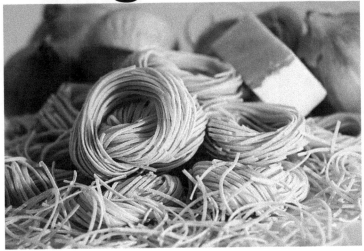

The Ultimate Healthy Lifestyle Guide with Quick, Easy and Fuss-Free Recipes, a Cookbook for Busy People and the Whole Family: Get Healthy, Lose Weight, and Feel Great!

Alice Louise Bayless

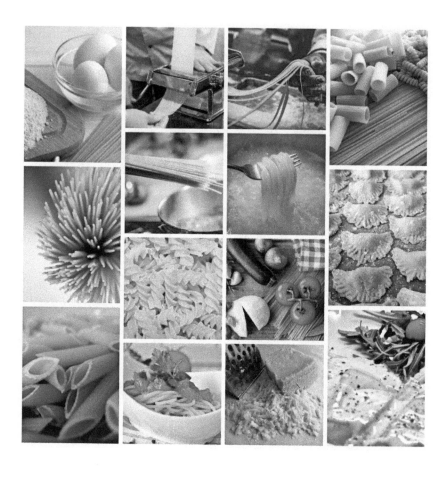

Table of Contents

    Gluten-Free Thai Chicken Soup
    Gluten-Free Golden Yam Brownies
    Gluten-Free White Bread for Bread Machines
    Gluten-Free Yellow Cake
    Perfect Gluten-Free Peanut Butter Cookies
    Gluten-Free Irish Soda Bread
    Delicious Gluten-Free Pancakes
    Gluten-Free Chocolate Cake with Semi-Sweet Chocolate Icing
    Amazing Gluten-free Layer Bars
    Gluten Free Macadamia Pie Crust
    Perfect Cashew and Peanut Butter Gluten-free Cookies

Gluten Free Chocolate Cupcakes
Garbanzo Bean Chocolate Cake (Gluten Free!)
Golly Gee Gluten-Free Pancakes
Gluten-free Peanut Butter Cookies
Gluten-free Mexican Wedding Cakes
Alison's Gluten Free Bread
Gluten-Free Pie Crust with LIBBY'S® Famous Pumpkin
Pie Filling
Chocolate Chip Cookies (Gluten Free)
Gluten-Free Fudge Brownies
Gluten-Free Orange Almond Cake with Orange Sauce
Dairy and Gluten-Free 'Buttermilk Pancakes'

Introduction

A lifestyle that is healthy and promotes a good quality of life is important.As a parent, it is also one of the best gifts you can give to your children. Food is a necessity for our bodies to thrive but we live in a society were eating habits have moved in the wrong direction.

A lack of time, a lack of information, and the availability of processed foods has resulted in obesity, increased health risks, and reduced lifespan. Thesenegative outcomes can make life difficult due to reduced energy, not being as alert, and an array of potential health problems.

If you are interested in making positive changes for yourself and for your household, consider the gluten free living option. You may be saying you are too busy for gluten free diet programs or that you will be limited in the foods you can buy.

However, this doesn't have to be the case. There are plenty of recipes and variety that are easy to make. There are more restaurants and grocery stores today that offer gluten free options than in the past. This is a lifestyle change that you will find there is a great deal of support surrounding and that makes it possible to successfully incorporate.

Until now, you may not have paid too much attention to gluten. Yet it is in so many of the foods that the average person eats without thinking twice about doing so. It seems to be everywhere you look now that you are making the effort to exclude it from your diet.

Instead of focusing on that negative fact though, focus on the positive changes you are going to make and the opportunity that you have to improve your overall well-being. As you learn more about gluten free products you can make better choices that help you.

Initially, a gluten free lifestyle may seem too hard to implement, but it doesn't have to be. Here, you will get the information you need about why you can live healthier and happier with this type of diet. You will find out methods for shopping and eating out that make it easier.

By eliminating the myths and sticking to the facts you can formulate your plan of action. You will get information about recipes, support, and the health benefits. As you read through the materials, you will be motivated to embrace such changes and you will have the methods to do so!

Not everyone out there is ready to act with a gluten free diet, and that is okay. Freedom of choice is very important. If you feel it is right for you than don't worry about what other people think. If you are friendly as you explain your reasons and while talking to those in a restaurant that are serving you then it isn't out of line at all.

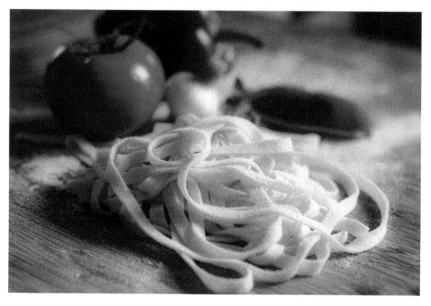

In 2010, various research companies including the National Restaurant Association and American Culinary Federation named gluten free as one of the top food priorities to consider for their establishments. They realizedthis was more than a passing trend.

For millions of people, it has become a lifestyle choice

that they engage in every single day. Are you ready to join them? It seems like all of the doors are wide open at this point when it comes to overall opportunity. The barriers that used to be in place such as limited products that were gluten free and a lack of information have been slowly removed.

Gluten problems can affect people of all ages, including children. There is no indication that any race or gender is more likely to be affected by it than others. The sooner that the problem is identified though the better.

Many adults develop this problem as they get older and there are a multitude of reasons why. There is nothing you can do to prevent it though as it is a genetic factor. You can take action though to live a good quality of life though in spite of the situation.

Chapter 1- Wheat and Celiac Disease, The Downside of Gluten

Wheat has been around for thousands of years. It's easy to grow and quite nutritious. It was probably one of the first food items our forefathers gathered to feed themselves. Wheat was truly life- giving.

For all these thousands of years, the whole grain kernel was ground and used to bake bread or prepare cereals. Fresh, whole grain has always been a part of our diet without being harmful to our health.

It's not until the 1960s and 70s that people began to realize that the wheat they are consuming is making them sick.

What happened? Have our bodies changed? No. It's the wheat we have relied on for thousands of years that has been changed and twisted into something our forefathers wouldn't recognize.

Industrialization has been good to mankind, but it hasn't always been kind to the food we consume.

Let's start with white flour, the first food that we would call "processed." In 1870, the steel roller mill allowed wheat to be separated to refine the wheat into a white powder. "White" flour was considered fancy.

So, to meet consumer demand, white flour was produced en masse, and the rest of the kernel, the nutritious part, was tossed aside. Within 10 years, all flour was white and seriously lacking in nutrients. Ten years was all the time it took to change thousands of years of nourishment into something "fancy" and lacking in many nutrients.

That was only the beginning, however. By the 1950s, technology once again let us "improve" our wheat. New techniques allowed for genetically-altered seeds, fertilizers, and harmful pesticides to increase wheat production. Again, everyone rejoiced. More wheat for everyone! Cake for one and all!

While the production of wheat increased, its nutritional value was being mangled into something unrecognizable. At the same time, inflammations and immune diseases were being linked directly to this new, "improved" wheat.

Anyone who believes that gluten-free is just a modern phase is half- right. It is indeed something new and modern. But it is not a phase. An increasing number of people are suffering from the effects of modern wheat and refined flour.

The degree can vary – from a bit of wheat sensitivity to

greater intolerance to celiac disease, which is the inability to process any amount of wheat due to problems in the small intestines. Especially in the case of celiac disease, the digestive system views gluten as invaders and reacts accordingly. As it tries to attack these toxins, the lining of the gut itself can become damaged, resulting in leaks, inflammation, and other problems.

Serious gastrointestinal problems are the result.

The number of people diagnosed with celiac disease has quadrupled in the past 50 years. One percent of the population suffers from celiac disease, and the number is rising. Wheat sensitivity affects up to 8 percent of the population. It is obvious that new "improved" wheat is making people sick.

In studies comparing modern, "improved" wheat to old wheat (called Einkorn), it was found that the old wheat had no harmful effects at all. No one who consumed unrefined wheat suffered any ill side effects or gastrointestinal problems. The same studies showed that modern wheat can affect our autoimmune system in harmful ways, leading to celiac disease and allergies.

People who are not allergic to modern wheat can still suffer. A 2013 study had healthy participants eat either new or old wheat for two months. The group that consumed the old wheat found their cholesterol level had decreased and their level of potassium and magnesium had increased. The opposite was true of the group given new wheat.

It is important to distinguish between gluten sensitivity and celiac disease, although they can have the same symptoms. Gluten sensitivity results in feelings of fatigue, bloating, diarrhea, nausea, and headaches. Many people don't even associate those feeling with wheat, so it's critical that doctors ask the right questions and test for wheat allergy.

People diagnosed with celiac disease suffer from identical symptoms, but the problem is more specifically defined. The gluten attacks the inflammatory system and can damage the small intestine. Inflammation is linked with a myriad of problems, such as heart disease, Alzheimer's, diabetes, and others.

The role of gluten itself is still being studied. What is clear, however, is that this modern, improved wheat is causing some serious illness. While wheat can be found almost everywhere, it is most commonly used in breads, cakes, cookies, pasta, creamed soups, sauces, cereal, and some salad dressings.

Rye wheat can be found in rye breads, beer, and some cereals.

Of course, wheat can be found in many other hidden places, and we will discuss this in much greater detail.

What is clear is that people who have eliminated wheat and gluten from their diet feel better and become healthier. With anyone suffering from celiac disease going gluten-free is a necessity. For others, it is a choice in an effort to enjoy increased health.

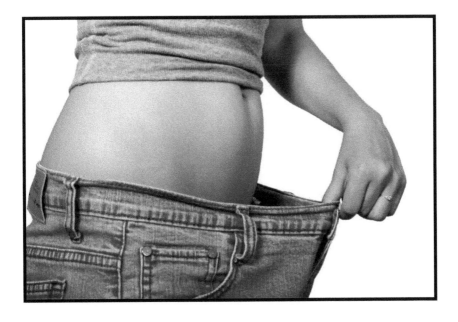

Most people also chose a gluten-free diet in order to lose

weight. A diet filled with breads, cakes, and noodles is high in carbohydrates and will very likely pack on the pounds. The reason for that is that refined wheat can cause a sugar spike. That means you use sugar for fuel while fat just gets stored and piled up. People find losing weight by cutting refined flour to be much easier and quicker.

Celiac disease can run in families and can be hereditary. People with parents or grandparents who have suffered from celiac disease have a 1 in 10 chance of becoming grain-intolerant.

Chapter 2 - Emotional Obstacles to Having Celiac Disease

A diagnosis of celiac disease can seem overwhelming. It's perfectly okay to feel upset. Celiac disease is serious, and it needs to be handled. You will undoubtedly feel shock at the diagnosis. Your first reaction may be denial. This can't be happening to you! All you can feel is a crushing frustration and anger at the unfairness of it all. These are perfectly normal reactions. There is no reason for you to deny your emotions. Feel whatever you need to feel. After all, this diagnosis will change a large part of your life.

At some point, you need to reach acceptance. You've been feeling sick and miserable for so long, you want to feel better. This is your chance. So, it up to you to become determined and deal with the situation.

Make no mistake. This may not be easy, especially if the decision to go gluten-free isn't your own. Here is why celiac disease can be such a difficult diagnosis to accept:

1. So many of our social interactions revolve around food. You have every right to wonder how this will change once you go gluten- free.

2. Family and friends may not understand your situation. Perhaps some of them tell you to just get over yourself. You may be accused of having an eating disorder. "It's just toast and scrambled eggs. Eat, for heaven sakes!" This lack of support just makes a difficult situation harder.

3. Knowing you'll need to give up some of your favorite can produce understandable anxiety. There is truth in the term "comfort food." Certain foods do comfort us. After your diagnosis, you realize your options will be limited. You have certain favorite dishes that you may not be able to enjoy anymore. It feels like losing a friend.

4. You will need to make some changes in your life. Depending on how well you react to change, that, too, can bring on anxiety.

5. You will have to follow new rules, and that isn't always easy. You used to be in control of your eating habits. Now you have to follow someone's rules!

6. There is no known cure for celiac disease. All you

can do is alleviate the symptoms by changing your eating habits. Yes, celiac is something you'll have to live with forever.

7.   Everyone around you is munching on Oreo cookies and devouring hamburger buns. You feel alone and isolated.

8.   A major problem for celiac sufferers is that they develop a gluten-free lifestyle, stick to it, and feel so much better after a while. That's when the rumbling in the brain can start. "I'm fine now. I can have that slice of pizza or cookie." "Grandma prepared this especially for me. I have to eat it." This can be one of the most difficult periods you'll have to with. You're so tempted … just one slice.

It's crucial to resist temptation. You're feeling better because you've eliminated gluten from your diet. Remember how miserable you felt before your new diet. Don't reverse the course that will force you to start over. You're exactly where you want to be. Keep going.

When You Are Tempted to Cheat
Sometimes, the urge to cheat – just a little bit – can be

overwhelming. This is especially true when special occasions arise. So many of our holiday memories are tied to food.

The problem is, there is no such thing as cheating "a little" when you have celiac disease. Even a minuscule amount of gluten can affect the immune system. So, it's not a matter of just one bite." For someone with celiac disease, any bite is a bite too many. Even people who are "only" gluten-sensitive can be severely affected by a small amount of it.

Gluten may cause the gut to leak from the small intestine, which can cause toxins to spread into the body and cause inflammations.

Consider seriously if mom's delicious stack of pancakes is worth this. This book is intended to help you make good choices.

The most serious case of cheating is done by gluten-sensitive people who don't show immediate negative symptoms. They may continue cheating, and gut is being damaged, although they don't know it until their autoimmune system is adversely affected. If you have been exposed to gluten, get a lab test before the damage caused become irreversible.

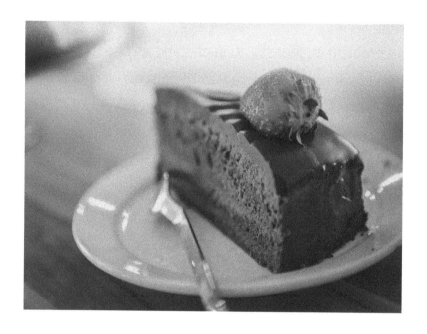

Cravings can pop up at any time. They can be difficult to handle, but you are in control. Like an alcoholic, take it one day at a time. You may want that piece of cake more than life itself at this moment. Just get through the moment. Walk away, if possible. Understand that the craving won't be as severe the next day. We repeat: handle cravings one day at a time and remain in control.

You also need to understand what foods trigger your cravings. Is it going to mom's house and having her prepare all of your childhood favorites? Is going out with friends for pizza too difficult to handle?

If you can't avoid the triggers (you really can't avoid mom), learn to handle them. Talk to mom about celiac disease and how to prepare gluten-free options; or bring your own. Discover pizza parlors with gluten-free selections and convince your friends to go there. Remember, cheating is always a choice. Make good choices for yourself.

Taking Control of Your Emotions

Let's not fool ourselves. Knowing you are suffering from celiac disease can cause bouts of blues and depression. When you start feeling down, it's time to elevate your emotions instead of obsessing on food. Following are some ways to feel better and enjoy a higher quality of life.

1. Depression can make you withdraw, but you need to reach out. Have at least one person you can talk to about what you are going through without worrying about judgments being made. This can be a parent, sibling, best friend, someone else who has celiac disease, or a professional. Just feeling understood can lift your spirits tremendously.

2. Instead of withdrawing, become more involved with people. Reach out to someone who is going through a rough time. Find a worthwhile association where you can volunteer and make a difference. Everyone is dealing with something. Knowing that will make you feel less alone.

3. While a pet won't replace other people, it can help you feel less alone.

4. Discover a new hobby or interest to get your mind off food. Taking a class, joining a gym, becoming involved in your community can be very energizing. Life has too much to offer to make it all about food.

5. If certain people are unsupportive of your situation or perhaps actually accusing you of overreacting, consider whether these people should remain in your life? What exactly are they adding to it?

6. Remove as much stress from your life as possible. Consider practicing meditation for half an hour daily. Just find a comfortable seat, close your eyes, and focus on your breath as you inhale and

exhale. This will relax your mind and spirit.

7.   Nature seems to be the best medicine of all. If you live in a city, find a park and walk around, enjoying what nature has to offer. Take a walk during your lunch hour. If you live in the country, communing with nature is even easier. It is true that sunshine will boost your day.

Chapter 3 - What is Gluten Free Living?

Gluten is a type of protein that is found in various foods including rye, barley, and wheat. While most of us take for granted being able to digest this protein that isn't the case for millions of others. Instead, their body struggles with it every time they consume any gluten.

There are some individuals that have an adverse reaction to gluten so they must eliminate it from their body. Their body will actually fight digesting it as it is deemed as the enemy and the body is ready to attack. This is why it can lead to nutritious deficiencies and also to chronic fatigue. The body isn't able to use the nutrients taken in and so much energy is spent fighting the gluten.

However, many people decide to make such a change in order to feel better and to promote longevity. Many popular celebrities talk about their gluten free diet and that tends to get the attention of the average person as well.

Gluten free living means you no longer consume the foods that contain gluten in them. You do need to make sure you watch out for cross contamination issues that can occur. For example, oats don't have gluten in them but due to the way they are processed and packaged they should be assumed to have gluten in them unless the packaging for that particular product specifically states otherwise.

You will still get to consume a wide variety of foods though which is very important. No one wants to feel like they are strictly limited to just a few choices for their meals. There are gluten free main courses, side dishes, and even desserts you can enjoy. The food tastes great too so you aren't going to be settling for bland options or food that you have to force yourself to consume.

It is also important to know that a proper gluten free lifestyle offers your body the vitamins, minerals, and fiber that you need on a daily basis. A large portion of your diet will include fresh fruits and vegetables. If you already like to eat fruits and vegetables then this is going to be an easier lifestyle change for you than you might have thought.

They also offer your body powerful antioxidants to help remove toxins from your body. You will feel satisfied rather than hungry, provide your body with fuel, and have energy for your daily routine and exercise.

You may be fearful at first about a diet that is free from

gluten but you will be very happy with the choices out there. You will find a variety of great foods and you can even have cake and other delicious items made with flour alternatives.

See your Doctor

It isn't recommended to self diagnose when it comes to a gluten problem. You should consult with your doctor to have the correct testing done. Some of the symptoms of gluten problems can be the same as other forms of health problems so it is important to get a professional diagnosis.

Continue to eat the way you normally would though when you are scheduled for the testing. If there is no gluten in your body then the blood work isn't going to be able to determine that it is the core of the problem (if 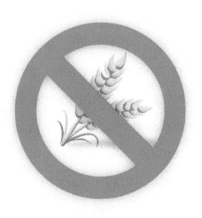 indeed it is)! If your blood work shows that there is a problem then you can remove the gluten.

Of course if you are making the change because you want to and not because of a medical concern then you can make the change when youare ready. Either use up the items you have in your home with gluten or toss them out and make a fresh break from it. Many people find tossing those items in the trash is quite empowering!

The outreach in place for this type of testing has significantly grown in the past couple of years. Part of the education process involves getting more doctors to prescribe such testing for their patients. By 2019 the goal is to successfully diagnose as many cases as possible so that children and adults with a gluten concern aren't slipping through the cracks and increasing the risk of serious health problems.

Some individuals will still notice they have some symptoms even after they switch to a gluten free diet. This can be due to the severity of their condition. It can also be due to the damage that has occurred for the small intestine. While the small intestine is healing itself, your doctor may recommend that you take dietary supplements in order if malnourishment has occurred.

Many individuals that are changing to a gluten free diet aren't getting the amount of certain vitamins that their body needs. Your doctor may recommend a supplement to increase the amount of Vitamin B, iron, zinc, or calcium. If such supplements are recommended take them until your doctor feels you no longer need them.

Household Items to Watch for

Most people have the understanding that gluten is only found in foods that you consume. However, there are some household items that may containit so you need to be diligent in looking at them too. Here are the most common ones that you need to take a very close look at before you use them again. It will depend on the brand so you need to read the label:

- Chapstick
- Glue
- Gum
- Medicines (Including over the counter, herbal remedies, andprescriptions)
- Toothpaste

Chapter 4 - Why is Gluten Free Living a Good Idea?

Some individuals have no choice but to follow a gluten free lifestyle due to the way their bodies process it. Celiac disease is a type of autoimmune disorder that results in the body rejecting gluten instead of processing it. The gluten is seen as a toxin to their bodies and it can create very serious health problems.

The severity of the reaction can vary based on the individual and the amount of gluten that they consume. A gluten allergy is extremely common, but it is very rarely diagnosed. Today, more people are informed about the symptoms and more medical professionals are testing for it.

This is why the number of children with sensitivity to gluten is being identified. There are adults that have struggled with their health for their entire life though because this gluten problem was never addressed. The sooner that a person is diagnosed though the sooner changes to their diet can be implemented.

It is believed that 1 in 133 people have some form of Celiac disease. The problem is that when they are consuming gluten their small intestine is being damaged. This creates problems with the small intestine successfully absorbing nutrients that the body needs. Some reports indicate approximately 83% of the cases though aren't diagnosed.

Celiac disease is genetic so if anyone in your family has it then your risk increases. Some individuals have several symptoms and others don't have any at all. There are more than 300 possible symptoms that can occur, but these are the most common:

- Abdominal pain
- Anemia
- Bloating
- Bone pain
- Chronic fatigue
- Depression
- Diarrhea
- Fertility problems
- Gas
- Headaches
- Weight changes

Children may have some other symptoms that develop

including:

- Behavioral changes
- Dental enamel damage
- Distended abdomen
- Failure to gain weight or height at their percentile

In order to confirm such a diagnosis, blood work is completed. If it comes back positive, than a biopsy of the small intestine will be done to see if the lining has been damaged as well as the degree of any damage that has occurred. There is no cure for Celiac disease other than to follow a gluten free diet.

Doing so allow the small intestine to heal and in time it can allow a person to make a full recovery. Their body will start being able to use the nutrients that they consume for better overall health. The problem will get worse if dietary changes aren't made including malnutrition, osteoporosis, neurological problems, and Lymphoma.

Request testing for you and your children if possible because so many people go undiagnosed with this type of problem. If you think this could be the issue, don't want until your doctor brings up the idea of the testing. Ask your family members too in order to determine if there is a high chance of itoccurring for you or your child.

Some individuals develop Dermatitis Herpetiformis, often referred to as DH, which is a type of Celiac disease that affects the skin. In order to diagnosis it blood work and a skin biopsy are conducted. The only cure for it is also a gluten free diet.

Such a test is a good ideas as this type of skin problem is often mistaken for Eczema. It can be very frustrating when the medication for Eczema is given but the condition either stays the same or gets worse. Until the diet ischanged then the skin isn't going to clear up.

Many people make the choice to have a gluten free diet even though they don't have the disease. Some have a family history of many health problems and they are being as proactive as possible to reduce the risk of serious health concerns for them personally.

If you decide to make this your lifestyle due to your own personal beliefs, you need to stand up for it. Don't let others that don't agree with you or that don't understand your decision to create problems or doubts for you. Not everyone in your life will be supportive about it but the majority of people will.

A gluten free lifestyle isn't something to be shy about, to

be ashamed of, or that you need to hide. It may be different from other people and the food choices they make but that is okay. It is about doing what is right for you and for your family in this regard so don't succumb to peer pressure.

Parents try to do all they can to create a world for their children that is fair, that is fun, and that is rewarding. Yet there can be issues with children that society as a whole isn't kind about. For example, children that have ADD or ADHD or those with Autism.

As the parent of a child with those types of issues, it can be exhausting. It can be hard for you and your partner to deal with on a daily basis. You may feel like you have been isolated by your friends and family because of it. Not giving up on your child though is important.

Some parents have found that their child did significantly improve by removing gluten from their diet. This was a better option or them than medicating their child. When there are behavior issues that aren't explained, it is definitely worth trying a gluten free diet for a few months andmonitoring the behavior of your child.

If you see improvements, then that is encouraging and

you should continue the diet. It could make a huge difference in the happiness of your child, in the dynamics of your household, and even how your child is accepted socially.

There are a few studies out there that indicate a gluten free diet can be a way to reduce symptoms of other forms of autoimmune deficiencies too. This includes:

- Cystic Fibrosis
- Multiple Sclerosis
- Thyroid Disease

Such information is very encouraging because it can be very upsetting to deal with the symptoms of these autoimmune deficiencies. They can create pain, fatigue, and other symptoms that affect every element of a person's life. If changing to a gluten free diet can make these health problems more manageable, isn't it worth it to consider?

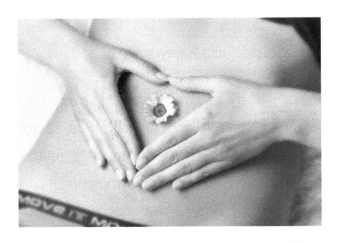

Other individuals have taken on a gluten free lifestyle due to having a child or partner that needs to follow such a diet plan. It is certainly easier to create meals that everyone in the household can consume rather than making something different from the person that can't have gluten. Plus, if a parent has a gluten related issue that it is very possible children in the household will at some point. Teaching them a healthier way of eating from an early age is important.

There are people that choose not to consume gluten because they feel better removing it from their diet. While they didn't test positive for Celiac disease, they may have some sort of wheat allergy. They may have an intolerance or sensitivity to gluten.

They often have gas or bloating when they consume it so they have removed if from their diet to be more comfortable. They don't have damage to the small intestine due to the gluten but they just feel better overall bynot consuming it anymore.

No one wants to try to get through their day continually with bloating and gas. It can make it hard to focus on work, social activities, and even intimate relationships. With the anxiety gone about such symptoms, it can give a person a refreshing and upbeat outlook about life that was missing before.

Weight loss and weight maintenance has also been a reason to stopconsuming gluten. The craving for sweets can make it hard to stick to a good diet plan but many people find they don't have cravings after a few weeks of a gluten free diet.

They also find that they lose weight and keep it off because they are no longer reaching for foods that have empty calories or snacks that are processed. Such changes can also do wonders for the amount of energy a person has.

Many people feel that they have been on a losing course for weight loss forquite some time. They don't have the willpower to stick with a program that is restricting them and they really shouldn't. Fad diets may be very popular but they are really just setting people up to fail. Many people find that they can stick with a gluten free diet and that they do lose weight.

There are a few reasons for that to occur. As previously mentioned, the cravings go away and that makes selecting healthier choices easier. Reducing the amount of processed foods that are consumed means that there is less harmful carbs that the body will store as fat. There is also less sugar intake that will be stored as fat.

The increased energy with this lifestyle also gives someone that help them may need to really exercise. They may have had a hard time doing so before but now they have both the energy and the motivation to stick with a plan of action. As they feel better and their mood improves it becomes a path that they would like to continue going down.

The verdict is still out there by the experts though regarding recommending the gluten free diet for weight loss. Since it can't be proven without in depth and time consuming studies you won't find doctor's that readily recommendit. However, you will find plenty of people that state it was the change that allowed them to feel great and to drop the pounds when nothing else worked.

If you have hit a point where you feel like losing weight is a lost cause, you may wish to give this type of lifestyle a try for a 90-day period. If you find that you feel better, you have more energy, and that you have lost weight then it is an option to continue with it.

Regardless of your reason for deciding to follow a gluten free diet – by necessity or by choice – it doesn't have to be hard and it doesn't have to be time consuming. It doesn't mean that you have a huge grocery bill or that you can't enjoy going out to eat.

If you travel often, you may be worried but you can use the internet to help you find great menu choices and restaurants anywhere you may go that offer gluten free selections. You have the ability to make this work for you and all of the information you need is at your fingertips!

Children and Gluten Free Diets

If your child is following a gluten free diet – by necessity or by yourparenting choice – talk to them about it. It is amazing what children can learn even from an early age about making good food choices. Explain to them the importance of their food choices.

Let them know that if they are in doubt about what they can eat then they should refrain from consuming it until they get approval from an adult. Make sure your child's gluten diet is well known when they go to stay with a friendtoo. You can talk to the parent's in advance to make accommodations.

Offer to send a gluten free meal and snacks so that they don't feel obligated to buy special items for your child to be a guest in their home. This also reduces the risk that they may not properly follow labeling due to not having enough information to make the right choices.

At the other end of that spectrum, think about elderly individuals you maybe responsible for. If you make their meals or they are in an assisted care facility they may need a gluten free diet plan. Make sure anyone that is in charge of their care understands what they can eat and what they can't.

Exercise

It is very important to point out that daily exercise is important for people of all ages. Taking part in a gluten free diet is a step in the right direction for overall health, losing weight, and maintaining a healthy body weight. Exercise still needs to be a part of the daily routine. Many individuals didn't exercise enough before due to their diet.

They continually felt fatigued and sluggish so it was hard for them to take part in working out. Once they changed to a gluten free diet though they found that they were able to benefit from the additional energy. They were energetic all day long too without peaks and valleys in there that once required a sugar intake as a pick me up.

Talk to your doctor about starting any new exercise program. Keep in mind that if you make too many changes at once to your lifestyle it will be hard tostick with it. Focus on the dietary changes and becoming familiar with what you can eat and what you can't first.

Then as your energy level increases and you are getting comfortable with your dietary changes you can look at the exercise plan. Find forms of exercise you can take part in that are at your fitness level. You should also take part in forms of exercise that you will enjoy so you will stick with them.

Chapter 5 - Shopping for Food & Eating Out

Planning your meals is an important part of a gluten free lifestyle. It reducesthe need for you to make an unhealthy choice because you are pushed for time. Plan your snacks too so that you always have something you can reach for when you get hungry. You don't have to be overwhelmed by the task of going to the grocery store though.

There are more stores that offer gluten free products than you may realize. The demand for them as well as the variety of options continues to grow all the time. You can go online to find out where to shop locally for those items you want. If you aren't finding enough selection, talk to the manager.

They may be willing to add a few gluten free items to what they normally stock if customers ask for it. Studies show that as of 2012, approximately 15% of customers were shopping for only gluten free products. Up to 25% were buying products gluten free as they have scaled down on the volume of gluten that they consume.

The predictions from U.S. News and World Report is that this percentage is only going to continue to climb in the future. Retailers that sell groceries are certainly going to be paying attention to this information as well and preparing the shelves in their stores to meet that demand.

Being well informed is important when you are shopping for gluten free products. Some of the common foods you may normally reach for to add to your basket contain gluten including:

- Bagels
- Cereal
- Crackers
- Pasta
- Pizza

Identifying what you can safely eat and what you can't is important so that you can be a great shopper. To help you feel better about all of this, focus on what you can eat and not what you are giving up.

Remember the many health benefits that you will gain when you start to feel your willpower slipping. The more you shop for gluten free items, the easier it becomes. Soon, it will be second nature for you when you enter the store.

Carefully Read Labels!

Different brands of products can contain gluten or not so you need to become familiar with the products out there. Don't be in a rush when you shop so that you can take all the time you need to read labels. Some products say gluten free and others say low gluten.

Fruits and Vegetables

Any fresh fruits and fresh vegetables that you see in the grocery store aren't processed and they are gluten free. You can buy sweet potatoes and white potatoes as they don't contain any gluten either. Both dry beans and peas are acceptable.

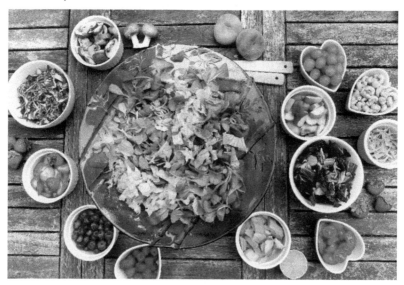

Dairy

Just about all of the milk and cheese that you will find at the grocery store are free of gluten. There are some exceptions though so you need to carefully read labels. Some processed cheese products have wheat in them and blue cheese does. If you buy plain yogurt there is no gluten. However, if you buy various flavors then there can be so always check the labels.

Meat, Fish, Pork, & Poultry

Look for lean cuts of meat, pork, and poultry. Only buy fresh fish and other forms of seafood. When you are looking at canned or frozen products in this category, many of them can contain gluten due to the processing. Always take the time to carefully read the labels. When possible, use fresh products instead of frozen or canned as they are better for you.

Grains

Select grains that are free of gluten. You will find that you can pick the varieties you like too. There are gluten free options with white, brown, and wild rice so your choice won't be limited.

Dining Out

When it comes to dining out, spend some time looking online to identify which restaurants offer you such dishes. This is very important if you are traveling and aren't familiar with the area. With the technology today, you can use your smartphone or a laptop to see what is available where you happen to be.

If you aren't able to do that, ask when you arrive about any gluten free foods that they may offer. Some locations are willing to make something special for you. With more restaurants trying to appease the needs of everyone it is possible they will work with you. Try to arrive at off peak times so they can provide you with personalized service.

There are some common items you can get though that would be fine. For example, order chicken or fish with a side of vegetables. You can also get abaked potato and a salad. You may want to ask what type of oil that fish or chicken is cooked in though as some of them do contain gluten.

There is a great deal of gluten in various marinades and sauces. If you aren't sure they are free of gluten it is best to avoid them. You can ask for them to be put on the side and most restaurants will be happy to comply.

Don't expect there to be gluten free bread or crackers though so make sureyou don't reach for them unless you are positive!

It is fine to consume champagne and wine as they are made from grapes. However, most beer is going to be off limits due to the grains they use to make them. You will find some gluten free beer offers though in many restaurants so it doesn't hurt to ask. You can also consider various forms ofmixed drinks.

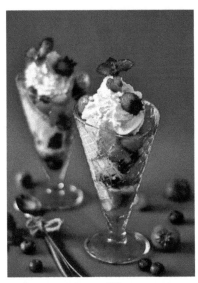

If dessert is something you just don't want to pass up, you aren't going to have to. There are some great choices in this category too. If the restaurant is gluten free friendly they may have flourless cake available. You can also consider sorbet, sherbet, fresh fruit, or ice cream. They are universal options so there is a very good chance they will be available.

Some labels on products aren't as clear as they should

be when it comesto determining if they contain gluten or not. If that is the case with aparticular product, err on the side of caution. Don't buy it and you can do some research at home about it. You can always buy that product on your next shopping trip if you do find it is actually free of gluten.

The more you are aware of what you can eat and what you shouldn't, the easier it is for you to shop and for your to dine out without stress or worry. See appendix 1 for a list to help you as you work to become more familiar with your options.

Chapter 6 – Tips For Recipes

It is a good idea to add the following items to your shopping list and to keep them on hand in your kitchen. They are commonly called for in gluten free recipes. You can also use them when you run low on food items for your menu to make something.

- Gluten free baking mix
- Gluten free crackers
- Gluten free bread crumbs
- Gluten free flour
- Gluten free snacks
- Guar Gum
- Quinoa
- Rice (brown or white depending on your preference)
- Xantham Gum

With these items you can also use some of your favorite recipes but with a gluten free value to them. It can be both fun and productive to get creative with those recipes. Here are some great tips for starting with such replacements:

- Binders – Use Xanthan Gum, Guar Gum, or gelatin.

- Breading – Wheat or gluten free bread crumbs or crushed potatochips.

- Flour – Use gluten free flour mix or cornstarch. There are plenty ofoptions to consider including amaranth and sorghum.

- Thickening – Use cornstarch or gluten free baking mix. For a sweetrecipe, use dry pudding mix.

The internet is a wonderful resource for finding various gluten free recipes to try. You will enjoy the new tastes and you will gain more confidence in this lifestyle choice as you are able to create meals you and your family love. You can also buy gluten free cookbooks, magazines, or exchange recipes with others that are also eating gluten free.

Here are some great ideas to get you started. Try some new recipes and create a file for those that you really like. As your file grows you can ensure lots of variety in your diet so you don't feel restricted or bored by eating the same thing over and over again.

Breakfast Ideas

Yogurt is a great option but make sure it is gluten free as many varieties aren't. Both Stonyfield and Chobani are certified by the Gluten Intolerant Group. You can use the yogurt as a basis for a delicious tasting smoothie too.

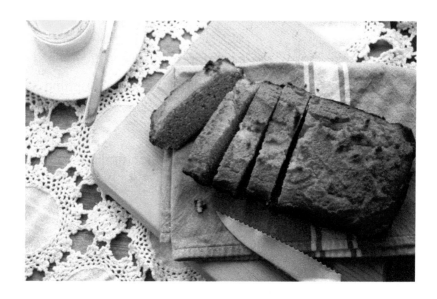

There are various brands of gluten free cereal by General Mills and Nature's Path. If you like hot cereal consider Cream of Buckwheat. There are also oats that are certified to be gluten free. Eggs that are fried or scrambled are a great way to start the day due to the amount of proteinthey offer.

Lunch Ideas

Lunch meat is a great choice for a convenient and gluten free option, but make sure it isn't processed. A salad can be a choice that works for you due to all of the vegetables. You have to be careful though as some of the cheese items and various dressings can have gluten in them.

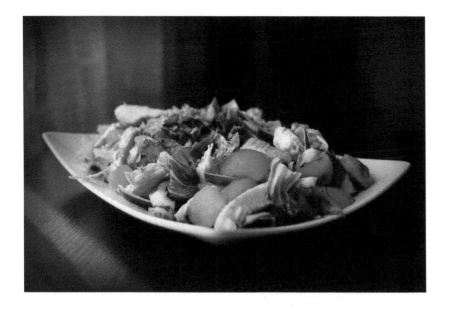

Nachos consisting of tortilla chips and some melted cheese that is gluten free is a change from your basic lunch and very appetizing. Peanut butter on gluten free bread is another great consideration.

Dinner Ideas

Lean cuts of meat including beef, pork, and poultry are great choices. You can also consume fresh fish or other seafood. Adding fresh vegetables and your choice of potatoes offers you a wonderful meal without gluten in no time at all. You can also replace the potatoes with your choice of glutenfree rice.

Snack Ideas

Gluten free snacks you can enjoy between meals will keep you on track. Cut up fresh fruit and vegetables so you can grab them and go. You can pack them to take in the car or to have at your desk while working.

There are plenty of types of cheese that don't contain gluten, and they are wonderful for snacking. They also help you to get your calcium. With certain flavors of cheese you need to be careful as they can have some gluten in them so always read the packaging. Kids seem to really enjoy those individually wrapped cheese sticks.

While you should only consume chips in moderation, they are also gluten free when it comes to many varieties including most of those offered by Frito Lay. For a lower calorie snack consider popcorn.

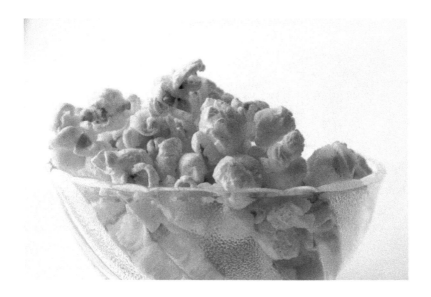

Make some hardboiled eggs and consume them when you need a snack. They will giveyou lots of energy.

Dessert Ideas

Both children and adults enjoy dessert, and you don't have to eliminate it due to a gluten free diet. Various brands of pudding are free of gluten and you will have a variety of flavors to pick from. Ice cream can also be a wonderful treat but you need to pay attention to the labels. So many ice cream varieties these days are packed with goodies so you need to pay attention to what is in there.

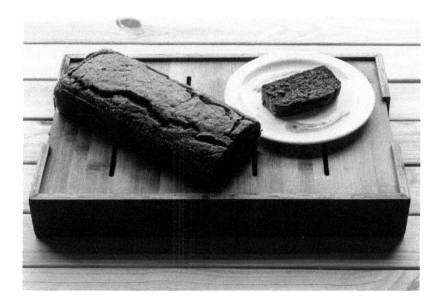

Cross Contamination

It is very important that you think about the risk of cross contamination in your own kitchen as well as those of others that prepare gluten free meals for you or your family. If the same tools are used to prepare such items as those that do have gluten then there can be some contamination.

Even a small amount of gluten can be dangerous to certain individuals so care has to be taken to prevent this. It is one more reason why changing the entire family to a gluten free diet may be the best option to consider.

Holidays

For many people, the holidays can be tough due to the restrictions of the diet. There can be parties to attend and various events where you have to be very careful about what you eat.

You may decide to make dinner at your own home and offer a gluten free meal for all. It is certainly an option to consider. Prepare yourself for the holidays and have a few items you can take along for snacks with you in case an event isn't gluten free friendly.

Chapter 7 - Support

Your decision to be gluten free is one you should feel proud of no matter why you have made that decision. It is a good idea to get a support system in place as soon as you can about it. Share with your family, friends, and co-workers about your lifestyle change and what it entails. You will be pleasantly surprised at the many people that support you and even think about making the change for their own household.

Tell your healthcare providers about such changes too if they haven'tmandated it due to a medical necessity. You will find that most medical professionals are very supportive of this type of dietary change.

Being well informed is important so you should consider magazines, books, and websites. However, you need to make sure you fully explore the credibility of such resources or you will end up with so much conflicting information it can make your head spin.

If you have questions, there are some very good organizations where you can direct your questions. They include the Celiac Disease Foundation and the Gluten Intolerance Group.

There are plenty of online forums where you can get support and meet newpeople. You may find it useful to be able to ask questions from those that are also going through similar changes in their lifestyle.

Being able to share recipes, to vent when you are discouraged, and even to be able to get some encouragement when you really need it is important. You can also offer support to others from time to time so it becomes a give and take.

Don't underestimate the value of this type of support as it helps to educate people about gluten free diets. The volume of the masses can also encourage more gluten free products in restaurants and grocery stores.

If you have children, make sure that their caregivers and teachers know they are on a gluten free diet. You may need to send your child with their lunch daily as the school or daycare lunch menu may not reflect thischoice.

You may need to provide snacks too but if you feel this is the right method for your household then your caregiver and the school should work with you. Check to see if there are any gluten free cooking classes offered in your community.

This can be a great way to learn some new cooking methods, try some delicious recipes, and make some terrific friends that you can count on to help you as you help them get used to these dietary changes. You may findworking with a dietician is useful as well.

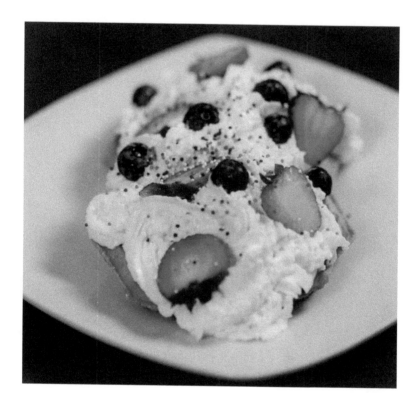

Chapter 8 – 22 Gluten Free Recipes

Below a list of 22 delicious Gluten Free Recipes:

- Gluten-Free Thai Chicken Soup
- Gluten-Free Golden Yam Brownies
- Gluten-Free White Bread for Bread Machines
- Gluten-Free Yellow Cake
- Perfect Gluten-Free Peanut Butter Cookies
- Gluten-Free Irish Soda Bread
- Delicious Gluten-Free Pancakes
- Gluten-Free Chocolate Cake with Semi-Sweet Chocolate Icing
- Amazing Gluten-free Layer Bars
- Gluten Free Macadamia Pie Crust
- Perfect Cashew and Peanut Butter Gluten-free Cookies
- Gluten Free Chocolate Cupcakes
- Garbanzo Bean Chocolate Cake (Gluten Free!)
- Golly Gee Gluten-Free Pancakes
- Gluten-free Peanut Butter Cookies
- Gluten-free Mexican Wedding Cakes
- Alison's Gluten Free Bread
- Gluten-Free Pie Crust with LIBBY'S® Famous

Pumpkin Pie Filling

- Chocolate Chip Cookies (Gluten Free)
- Gluten-Free Fudge Brownies
- Gluten-Free Orange Almond Cake with Orange Sauce
- Dairy and Gluten-Free 'Buttermilk Pancakes'

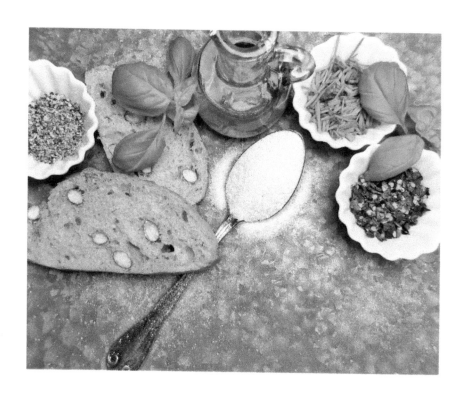

LET'S START!

Gluten-Free Thai Chicken Soup

Ingredients

1 tablespoon grapeseed oil
3 shallots, chopped
2 tablespoons chopped cilantro
4 cups chicken stock
2 (14 ounce) cans coconut milk
1 tablespoon agave nectar
1 (8 ounce) package crimini mushrooms, sliced
1 head broccoli, cut into florets
1 pound thinly sliced chicken breast meat
2 teaspoons red curry paste
3 tablespoons lime juice
3 tablespoons fish sauce

1/2 cup chopped fresh cilantro
2 serrano chile peppers, thinly sliced
1/4 cup chopped green onions
8 lime wedges

Directions

Heat the grapeseed oil in a large saucepan over medium heat. Cook and stir the shallots and 2 tablespoons chopped cilantro in the hot pan until the shallot has softened and turned translucent, about 4 minutes. Pour in the chicken stock, coconut milk, and agave nectar; bring to a simmer over medium-high heat. Once the broth reaches a simmer, strain through a mesh strainer into a clean saucepan; discard the shallot and cilantro.

Return the broth to a simmer; stir in the mushrooms and broccoli and cook until the broccoli becomes tender, about 4 minutes. Add the chicken and cook until no longer pink, stirring constantly. Stir the curry paste, lime juice, and fish sauce in a small bowl to dissolve the curry paste; mix into the simmering soup.

Ladle the soup into bowls and sprinkle with 1/2 cup cilantro, serrano peppers, green onions, and lime wedges to serve.

1

Gluten-Free Golden Yam Brownies

Ingredients

2 tablespoons dry egg replacer (such as Ener-G®)
1/2 cup water
1 1/2 cups sweet rice flour (mochiko)
1 1/2 teaspoons xanthan gum
1 teaspoon baking powder
1/2 teaspoon salt
1 cup vegan margarine (such as Earth Balance®)
1 cup packed brown sugar
1 cup turbinado sugar (such as Sugar in the Raw®)
2 teaspoons gluten-free vanilla extract
2 cups peeled and finely shredded yam

3/4 cup turbinado sugar (such as Sugar in the Raw®)
1/4 cup cornstarch
2 tablespoons vegan margarine (such as Earth Balance®), softened
2 tablespoons almond milk

Directions

Preheat an oven to 350 degrees F (175 degrees C). Grease a 9x13-inch baking dish.

Stir the egg replacer and water together in a small bowl until the powder is completely integrated. Stir the rice flour, xanthan gum, baking powder, and salt together in a separate bowl.

Beat 1 cup margarine, brown sugar, and 1 cup turbinado sugar with an electric mixer in a large bowl until light and fluffy. Add the egg replacer about 1/2 cup at a time, allowing each addition to blend into the butter mixture before adding the next. Add the vanilla extract with the last of the egg replacer. Pour the rice flour mixture into the batter, mixing until just incorporated. Fold the shredded yam into the batter, mixing just enough to evenly combine. Pour the batter into prepared pan.

Bake in the preheated oven until a toothpick inserted into the center comes out clean, about 30 minutes.

Stir 3/4 cup turbinado sugar, cornstarch, 2 tablespoons margarine, and almond milk together in a small bowl until smooth. Spread over the brownies while still warm; they will absorb some of the glaze. Serve warm.

2

Gluten-Free White Bread for Bread Machines

Ingredients

3 eggs
1 tablespoon cider vinegar
1/4 cup olive oil
1/4 cup honey
1 1/2 cups buttermilk, at room temperature
1 teaspoon salt
1 tablespoon xanthan gum
1/3 cup cornstarch
1/2 cup potato starch
1/2 cup soy flour
2 cups white rice flour
1 tablespoon active dry yeast

Directions

Place ingredients in the pan of the bread machine in the order recommended by the manufacturer.

Select the sweet dough cycle. Five minutes into the cycle, check the consistency of the dough. Add additional rice flour or liquid if necessary.

When bread is finished, let cool for 10 to 15 minutes before removing from pan.

3

Gluten-Free Yellow Cake

Ingredients

1 1/2 cups white rice flour
3/4 cup tapioca flour
1 teaspoon salt
1 teaspoon baking soda
3 teaspoons baking powder
1 teaspoon xanthan gum
4 eggs
1 1/4 cups white sugar
2/3 cup mayonnaise
1 cup milk
2 teaspoons gluten-free vanilla extract

Directions

Preheat oven to 350 degrees F (175 degrees C). Grease and rice flour two 8 or 9 inch round cake pans.

Mix the white rice flour, tapioca flour, salt, baking soda, baking powder and xanthan gum together and set aside.

Mix the eggs, sugar, and mayonnaise until fluffy. Add the flour mixture, milk and vanilla and mix well. Spread batter into the prepared pans.

Bake at 350 degrees F (175 degrees C) for 25 minutes. Cakes are done when they spring back when lightly touched or when a toothpick inserted near the center comes out clean. Let cool completely then frost, if desired.

4

Perfect Gluten-Free Peanut Butter Cookies

Ingredients

1/2 cup gluten free, casein free margarine
1/2 cup brown sugar
1/2 cup white sugar
1 egg
1/2 cup salted natural peanut butter
1/2 teaspoon baking soda
1 cup soy flour
1/4 cup tapioca flour
1/4 cup potato flour

Directions

Preheat the oven to 375 degrees F (190 degrees C).

In a medium bowl, cream together the margarine, brown sugar and white sugar until smooth. Mix in the egg and peanut butter. Combine the baking soda, soy flour, tapioca flour and potato flour; stir into the batter to form a dough. Roll teaspoonfuls of dough into balls and place them 2 inches apart onto ungreased baking sheets.

Bake for 8 to 10 minutes in the preheated oven. Allow cookies to cool on baking sheet for 5 minutes before removing to a wire rack to cool completely.

5

Gluten-Free Irish Soda Bread

Ingredients

1 1/2 cups white rice flour
1/2 cup tapioca flour
1/2 cup white sugar
1 teaspoon baking soda
1 teaspoon baking powder
1 teaspoon salt
1 egg
1 cup buttermilk

Directions

Preheat oven to 350 degrees F (175 degrees C). Grease a 9 inch round cake pan.

Combine the rice flour, tapioca flour, sugar, baking soda, baking powder, and salt in a large bowl. In a separate bowl, whisk together egg and buttermilk . Make a well in the center of the dry ingredients and pour in the wet. Stir just until the dry ingredients are moistened. Pour into the cake pan.

Bake for 65 minutes in the preheated oven, or until a toothpick inserted into the center comes out clean. Cool on a wire rack, for 10 minutes before removing from the pan. Wrap bread in plastic wrap or aluminum foil and let stand overnight for the best flavor.

6

Delicious Gluten-Free Pancakes

Ingredients

1 cup rice flour
3 tablespoons tapioca flour
1/3 cup potato starch
4 tablespoons dry buttermilk powder
1 packet sugar substitute
1 1/2 teaspoons baking powder
1/2 teaspoon baking soda
1/2 teaspoon salt
1/2 teaspoon xanthan gum
2 eggs
3 tablespoons canola oil
2 cups water

Directions

In a bowl, mix or sift together the rice flour, tapioca flour, potato starch, dry buttermilk powder, sugar substitute, baking powder, baking soda, salt, and xanthan gum. Stir in eggs, water, and oil until well blended and few lumps remain.

Heat a large, well-oiled skillet or griddle over medium high heat. Spoon batter onto skillet and cook until bubbles begin to form. Flip, and continue cooking until golden brown on bottom. Serve immediately with condiments of your choice.

7

Gluten-Free Chocolate Cake with Semi-Sweet

Ingredients

1/2 cup sorghum flour
1/2 cup tapioca flour
1/2 cup rice flour
1 cup cocoa powder, sifted
1 1/2 tablespoons xanthan gum
2 1/2 teaspoons baking powder
1 teaspoon baking soda
3/4 cup butter at room temperature
3/4 cup (packed) dark brown sugar
1 cup white sugar
3 eggs
2 egg yolks
2 teaspoons vanilla extract
1 1/2 cups buttermilk

5 ounces chocolate chips
1/2 cup sour cream
1/2 teaspoon vanilla extract
1 tablespoon heavy cream

Directions

Preheat oven to 350 degrees F (175 degrees C). Grease a 9x13 inch pan and set aside.

In a medium bowl, sift together the sorghum, tapioca, and rice flours with the cocoa powder, xanthan gum, baking powder, and baking soda.

In a large mixer bowl, cream the butter until light and fluffy. Slowly beat in the brown and white sugars; whip until fluffy. Beat in the eggs and egg yolks one at a time. Add the vanilla. On low speed, alternately combine the buttermilk with the flour mixture. Pour batter into prepared pan.

Bake in preheated oven for 30 to 35 minutes, or until a toothpick inserted into the center of the cake comes out clean. Cool in pan.

To make the icing, in the top of a double boiler over medium high heat, melt the chocolate chips (or use microwave). Remove from heat and cool until warm. Stir in the sour cream and vanilla; add heavy cream. Stir in additional heavy cream to make desired consistency. Once the cake is thoroughly cool, spread a thin layer of frosting over the top.

8

Amazing Gluten-free Layer Bars

Ingredients

7 ounces flaked coconut
1 cup butterscotch chips
6 ounces semisweet chocolate chips
8 ounces unsalted peanuts
1/2 cup sliced almonds
1 (14 ounce) can sweetened condensed milk

Directions

Preheat oven to 350 degrees F (175 degrees C). Generously grease one 13x9 inch baking pan.

Spread 2/3 of the flaked coconut evenly on the bottom of the baking pan. Sprinkle the butterscotch morsel, chocolate chips, and peanuts evenly over the coconut layer. Pour condensed milk evenly over the whole pan. Top with sliced almonds and remaining coconut . Bake for 20 minutes in the preheated oven. Cool completely before cutting into squares.

9

Gluten Free Macadamia Pie Crust

Ingredients

6 ounces macadamia nuts
2 eggs
1 1/2 cups soy flour

Directions

Preheat the oven to 350 degrees F (175 degrees C).

Place the macadamia nuts into the container of a food processor, and blend until they reach a peanut butter like consistency. Scrape out into a bowl, and stir in the eggs and soy flour until well blended.

Place the dough between two pieces of waxed paper, and roll out into about a 12 inch circle. Remove the top piece of waxed paper, and invert the dough into a 9 inch pie plate. Press into the bottom and up the sides. Remove any overhanging dough.

Bake for 5 minutes in the preheated oven, or until light golden brown. Use in any recipe calling for a prebaked pie crust.

10

Perfect Cashew and Peanut Butter Gluten-free

Ingredients

1/2 cup brown sugar
1/2 cup white sugar
1 egg
1/4 cup salted natural peanut butter
1/4 cup cashew butter
1/2 cup gluten free, casein free margarine
1/2 teaspoon baking soda
1/2 cup corn flour
1/2 cup tapioca flour
1/4 cup potato flour

Directions

Preheat oven to 350 degrees F (175 degrees C).

In a medium bowl, mix together the margarine, brown sugar, white sugar and egg until smooth. Stir in the peanut butter and cashew butter. Combine the baking soda, corn flour, tapioca flour, and potato flour; stir into the batter to form a dough. Roll the dough into teaspoon sized balls and place them 2 inches apart onto an ungreased cookie sheet.

Bake for 8 to 10 minutes in the preheated oven. Let cool on baking sheets for a few minutes before removing to wire racks to cool completely.

11

81

Gluten Free Chocolate Cupcakes

Ingredients

1 1/2 cups white rice flour
3/4 cup millet flour
1/2 cup unsweetened cocoa powder
1 teaspoon salt
1 teaspoon baking soda
1 tablespoon baking powder
1 teaspoon xanthan gum
4 eggs
1 1/4 cups white sugar
2/3 cup sour cream
1 cup milk
2 teaspoons vanilla extract

Directions

Preheat oven to 350 degrees F (175 degrees C). Grease two 12 cup muffin pans or line with paper baking cups.

In a medium bowl, stir together the rice flour, millet flour, cocoa, salt, baking soda, baking powder and xanathan gum. In a separate large bowl, beat the eggs, sugar, sour cream, milk and vanilla. Stir in the dry ingredients until smooth. Spoon the batter into the prepared cups, dividing evenly.

Bake in the preheated oven until the tops spring back when lightly pressed, 20 to 25 minutes. Cool in the pan set over a wire rack. When cool, arrange the cupcakes on a serving platter.

12

Garbanzo Bean Chocolate Cake (Gluten Free!)

Ingredients

1 1/2 cups semisweet chocolate chips
1 (19 ounce) can garbanzo beans, rinsed and drained
4 eggs
3/4 cup white sugar
1/2 teaspoon baking powder
1 tablespoon confectioners' sugar for dusting

Directions

Preheat the oven to 350 degrees F (175 degrees C). Grease and flour a 9 inch round cake pan.

Place the chocolate chips into a microwave-safe bowl. Cook in the microwave for about 2 minutes, stirring every 20 seconds after the first minute, until chocolate is melted and smooth. If you have a powerful microwave, reduce the power to 50 percent.

Combine the beans and eggs in the bowl of a food processor. Process until smooth. Add the sugar and the baking powder, and pulse to blend. Pour in the melted chocolate and blend until smooth, scraping down the corners to make sure chocolate is completely mixed. Transfer the batter to the prepared cake pan.

Bake for 40 minutes in the preheated oven, or until a knife inserted into the center of the cake comes out clean. Cool in the pan on a wire rack for 10 to 15 minutes before inverting onto a serving plate. Dust with confectioners' sugar just before serving.

13

Golly Gee Gluten-Free Pancakes

Ingredients

1 egg
1/4 cup apple juice
1 tablespoon unsalted butter, melted
1/4 cup amaranth flour
1/4 cup tapioca flour
3 tablespoons arrowroot flour
1/4 teaspoon ground cinnamon
1 pinch ground nutmeg
1/2 teaspoon wheat-free baking powder
1/4 teaspoon salt

Directions

In a medium mixing bowl, beat the egg with the apple juice and melted butter. Add the remaining ingredients and stir.

Heat a lightly oiled griddle or frying pan over medium high heat. Pour or scoop the batter onto the griddle, using approximately 1/4 cup for each pancake. Brown on both sides and serve hot. This batter must be used right away and can not sit and wait.

14

84

Gluten-free Peanut Butter Cookies

Ingredients

2 cups peanut butter
2 cups white sugar
4 eggs, beaten
2 cups semi-sweet chocolate chips (optional)
1 1/2 cups chopped pecans (optional)

Directions

Preheat oven to 350 degrees F (175 degrees C). Grease cookie sheet.

Combine peanut butter, eggs, and sugar and mix until smooth. Mix in chocolate chips and nuts, if desired. Spoon dough by tablespoons onto a cookie sheet.

Bake for 10 to 12 minutes or until lightly browned. Let the cookies cool on the cookie sheets for 5 to 10 minutes before removing.

15

Gluten-free Mexican Wedding Cakes

Ingredients

1/2 cup butter
1 teaspoon gluten free vanilla
extract
1 cup confectioners' sugar
1/2 cup white rice flour
1/4 cup cornstarch
1/4 cup tapioca flour
1/4 teaspoon unflavored gelatin
(optional)
1 cup chopped hazelnuts
1 cup chopped walnuts or
hazelnuts
confectioners' sugar for dusting

Directions

Preheat the oven to 350 degrees F (175 degrees C).

In a medium bowl, mix together the butter and vanilla until well blended. Sift together the confectioners' sugar, rice flour, cornstarch, tapioca starch and gelatin. Stir into the butter mixture until all of the dry ingredients have been absorbed. Mix in the ground hazelnuts and chopped hazelnuts. Form teaspoonfuls of dough into balls, and shape into crescents. Place cookies at least 2 inches apart onto ungreased cookie sheets.

Bake for 8 to 10 minutes in the preheated oven, until golden brown. For crispier cookies, reduce heat to 325 degrees F (165 degrees C), and bake slightly longer. When cookies have cooled completely, dust with additional confectioners' sugar.

16

Alison's Gluten Free Bread

Ingredients

1 egg
1/3 cup egg whites
1 tablespoon apple cider vinegar
1/4 cup canola oil
1/4 cup honey
1 1/2 cups warm skim milk
1 teaspoon salt
1 tablespoon xanthan gum
1/2 cup tapioca flour
1/4 cup garbanzo bean flour
1/4 cup millet flour
1 cup white rice flour
1 cup brown rice flour
1 tablespoon active dry yeast

Directions

Place ingredients in the pan of the bread machine in the order recommended by the manufacturer. Select cycle; press Start. Five minutes into the cycle, check the consistency of the dough. Add additional rice flour or liquid if necessary.

When bread is finished, let cool for 10 to 15 minutes before removing from pan.

17

87

Gluten-Free Pie Crust with LIBBY'S® Famous

Ingredients

Crust:
1 cup white rice flour
1/2 cup potato starch
1/2 cup tapioca flour
1/4 teaspoon salt
6 tablespoons cold butter, cut into small pieces
1 large egg, beaten
1 tablespoon apple cider or white vinegar
3 tablespoons ice water, or as needed

Filling:
1 1/2 cups granulated sugar
1 teaspoon salt
2 teaspoons ground cinnamon
1 teaspoon ground ginger
1/2 teaspoon ground cloves
4 large eggs
1 (29 ounce) can LIBBY'S® 100% Pure Pumpkin
2 (12 fluid ounce) cans NESTLE® CARNATION® Evaporated Milk
Whipped cream or topping (optional)

Directions

For Pie Crust: Combine rice flour, potato starch, tapioca flour and salt in medium bowl. Cut in butter with pastry blender or two knives until mixture is crumbly. Form well in center. Add egg and vinegar; stir gently with a fork until just blended. Sprinkle with water; blend together with a fork and clean hands until mixture just holds together and forms a ball. (Be careful not to add too much water as dough will be hard to roll.)

Shape dough into ball and divide in half. Cover one half with plastic wrap; set aside. Place remaining half on lightly floured (use rice flour) sheet of wax paper. Top with additional piece of wax paper. Roll out dough to 1/8-inch thickness. Remove top sheet of wax paper and invert dough into 9-inch deep-dish (4-cup volume) pie plate. Slowly peel away wax paper. Trim excess crust. Turn edge under; crimp as desired. Repeat with remaining half.

For Filling: Mix sugar, salt, cinnamon, ginger and cloves in small bowl. Beat eggs in large bowl. Stir in pumpkin and sugar-spice mixture. Gradually stir in evaporated milk. POUR into pie shells.

Bake in preheated 425 degrees F. oven for 15 minutes. Reduce temperature to 350 degrees F.; bake for 40 to 50 minutes or until knife inserted near center comes out clean. Cool on wire rack for 2 hours. Serve immediately or refrigerate. Top with whipped cream or topping before serving.

18

Chocolate Chip Cookies (Gluten Free)

Ingredients

3/4 cup butter, softened
1 1/4 cups packed brown sugar
1/4 cup white sugar
1 teaspoon gluten-free vanilla extract
1/4 cup egg substitute
2 1/4 cups gluten-free baking mix
1 teaspoon baking soda
1 teaspoon baking powder
1 teaspoon salt
12 ounces semisweet chocolate chips

Directions

Preheat oven to 375 degrees F (190 degrees C). Prepare a greased baking sheet.

In a medium bowl, cream butter and sugar. Gradually add replacer eggs and vanilla while mixing. Sift together gluten- free flour mix, baking soda, baking powder, and salt. Stir into the butter mixture until blended. Finally, stir in the chocolate chips.

Using a teaspoon, drop cookies 2 inches apart on prepared baking sheet. Bake in preheated oven for 6 to 8 minutes or until light brown. Let cookies cool on baking sheet for 2 minutes before removing to wire racks.

19

Gluten-Free Fudge Brownies

Ingredients

2/3 cup gluten-free baking mix (such as Bob's Red Mill All Purpose GF Baking Flour®)
1/2 cup cornstarch
1 cup white sugar
1 cup packed brown sugar
3/4 cup unsweetened cocoa powder
1 teaspoon baking soda
2 eggs, beaten
3/4 cup margarine, melted

Directions

Preheat oven to 350 degrees F (175 degrees C), and grease an 8x8 inch square baking dish.

Stir together the gluten-free baking mix, cornstarch, white sugar, brown sugar, cocoa powder, and baking soda in a bowl, sifting with a fork to remove lumps. Pour in the eggs and melted margarine, and mix with a large spoon or electric mixer on low until the mixture forms a smooth batter, 3 to 5 minutes. Scrape the batter into the prepared baking dish.

Place a sheet of aluminum foil on the oven rack to prevent spills as the brownies rise, then fall during baking. Bake until a toothpick inserted in the center of the brownies comes out clean, 40 to 45 minutes.

20

Gluten-Free Orange Almond Cake with Orange

Ingredients

3 eggs, separated
2/3 cup white sugar
1/4 cup rice flour
1 teaspoon ground cinnamon
1/2 cup orange juice
1 1/2 cups finely ground almonds
(almond meal)

2 tablespoons heavy cream
2 cups white sugar
1 cup orange juice
1 tablespoon grated orange zest
1/2 cup butter
4 egg whites

Directions

Preheat the oven to 325 degrees F (165 degrees C). Grease a 10 inch springform pan with cooking spray, and dust with rice flour.

In a large bowl, whip egg yolks with 2/3 cup of sugar until thick and pale using an electric mixer. This will take about 5 minutes. Stir in the rice flour and orange juice, then fold in the almond meal and cinnamon.

In a separate glass or metal bowl, whip 3 egg whites until they can hold a stiff peak. Fold into the almond mixture until well blended. Pour into the prepared pan, and spread evenly.

Bake for 35 to 40 minutes in the preheated oven, until a toothpick inserted into the center comes out clean. Cool in the pan on a wire rack. Run a knife around the outer edge of the cake to help remove it from the pan.

To make the orange sauce, cream together the butter and 2 cups of white sugar in a medium bowl. Stir in the cream, and place the dish over a pan of barely simmering water. Stir in orange juice and zest. Whip 4 egg whites in a separate bowl until soft peaks form. Fold into the orange sauce. Spoon over the cake and serve immediately.

Dairy and Gluten-Free 'Buttermilk Pancakes'

Ingredients

1 cup sweet rice flour
2 teaspoons baking powder
1/2 teaspoon baking soda
1/2 teaspoon ground cinnamon
(optional)
1/2 teaspoon salt
2 eggs, beaten
1 1/4 cups soy yogurt
1/4 cup rice milk
2 tablespoons vegetable oil

Directions

Sift the rice flour, baking powder, baking soda, cinnamon, and salt in a bowl. In another bowl, whisk together the beaten eggs, soy yogurt, rice milk, and oil, and pour into the flour mixture. Stir briefly just to combine.

Heat a lightly oiled griddle or frying pan over medium-high heat. Scoop about 1/4 cup of batter per pancake onto the heated griddle, and cook for 1 to 2 minutes, until bubbles appear on the surface. Flip the pancake and cook 1 to 2 minutes more, until the pancake is golden brown on both sides.

22

92

Chapter 9 - Conclusion

Depending on what you currently eat, changing to a gluten free lifestyle may be a moderate change or a significant change. With the right information, you can accept those changes and become well aware of what you can eat and what you need to steer clear of.

For many individuals, they find that they have already been consuming plenty of foods on this list. Increasing the volume of fresh fruits and vegetables that they consume while reducing the intake of processed foods is the best place to start. Take the changes one step at a time so that you can focus on them.

Educate yourself about the reasons why a gluten lifestyle is right for you and get support all around you where you can. Learn about the foods to eat, where you can shop locally, and even online providers that have free or low cost shipping on the items you can't find locally.

Find out about restaurants that offer gluten free meals as well as safe items you can get from standard restaurants. It is possible to live gluten free and to feel very good about your decision to do so. It doesn't have to be expensive and it doesn't have to be difficult.

The good news is that there is more awareness out there about it than in the past. More grocery stores and restaurants are embracing the needs of this sector of consumers. When it comes to what you eat, the choice is always yours.

However, many people in our society today don't eat what they should for their overall health and well-being. With a diet that consists of lots ofprocessed foods you open up the opportunity for serious health problems that can reduce your quality of life and also your overall lifespan.

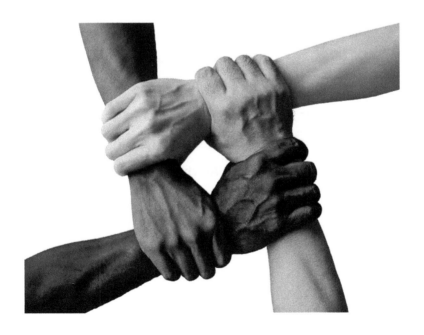

A gluten free diet isn't going to harm you like many fad diets will out there. This should be encouraging information if you are switching to this type of lifestyle because you want to rather than because you medically have to.

It is never too late to change your habits and start with a gluten free dietthat works well for you. This type of diet can work for your entire family and they won't feel like they are missing out on anything! Consider such changes an investment in your quality of life, your longevity, and your opportunity to really lead by example for your children!

It is estimated by 2015 that there will be more than $5 billion annually for sales of gluten free products. This isn't a passing trend, this is a lifestyle change and a way of life for many people. The possibilities continue to grow and that makes it easier to embrace this type of living without difficultyand without it being an expensive endeavor.

Appendix 1

You don't want to be second guessing yourself all the time when it comesto eating gluten free. Getting it right is easier than you think once you learn the foundation of all of it. Don't worry, it will get easier and you will spend less time reading labels and conducting research as time goes by.

You can consume any gluten free grain products including:

- Amaranth
- Buckwheat
- Corn flour
- Cornmeal
- Grits
- Millet
- Montina
- Quinoa
- Rice (brown, white, enriched, or basmati)
- Sorghum
- Soy
- Vegetable oil

Common Staples:

- Cheese (most blends but read the labels)
- Beans
- Butter
- Lean meats
- Legumes
- Fresh fruit
- Fresh seafood
- Fresh vegetables
- Margarine
- Milk
- Yogurt (plain, read the labels on flavored)

Any of the following various ingredients:

- Annatto
- Dextrose
- Glucose Syrup
- Lactose
- Lecithin

- Malodextrin (it can be consumed even when it is made from wheat)

- Oat gum

- Silicon Dioxide

- Starch

- Surcose

- Vinegar (except malt vinegar)

Lightning Source UK Ltd.
Milton Keynes UK
UKHW020755230421
382490UK00005B/54